Ruling Your World

*Discovering How To Activate & Build Your
Confidence To Overcome Low Self-Esteem*

Sensei Paul David

Copyright Page

Ruling Your World: Discovering How To Activate & Build Your Confidence To Overcome Low Self-Esteem, by Sensei Paul David

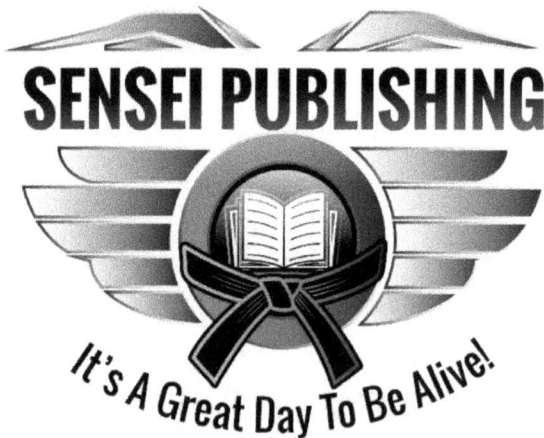

SENSEI PUBLISHING

It's A Great Day To Be Alive!

www.senseipublishing.com

@senseipublishing
#senseipublishing

Get/Share Our FREE All-Ages Mental Health Book Now!

FREE Self-Development Book for Every Family

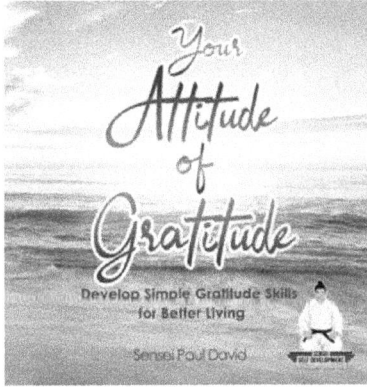

senseiselfdevelopment.senseipublishing.com

Click Below or Search Amazon for Another Book In This Series

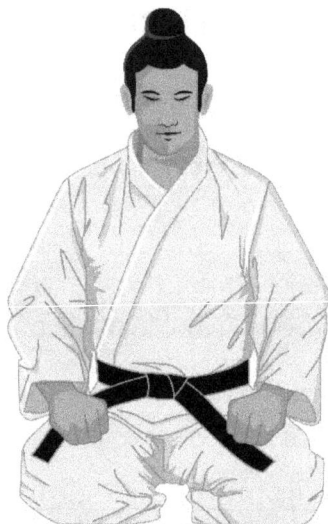

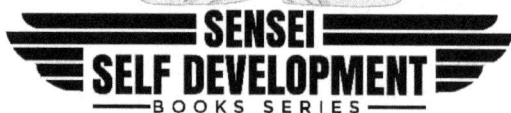

SENSEI SELF DEVELOPMENT
BOOKS SERIES

senseiselfdevelopment.senseipublishing.com

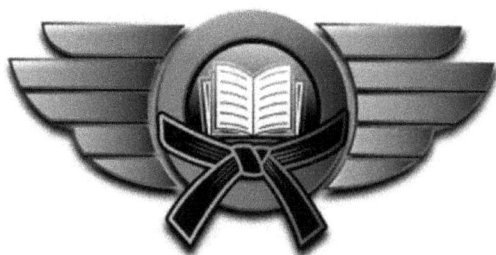

Join Our Publishing Journey!

If you would like to receive FUTURE FREE BOOKS and get to know us better, please click www.senseipublishing.com and join our newsletter by entering your email address in the pop-up box.

Follow Our Blog: senseipauldavid.ca

Follow/Like/Subscribe: Facebook, Instagram, YouTube: @senseipublishing

Scan the QR Code with your phone or tablet

to follow us on social media: Like / Subscribe / Follow

Thank You from The Author: Sensei Paul David

Before we dive in, I would like to thank you for picking up this book from among the many other similar books out there. Thank you for choosing to invest in my book. That means everything to me.

Now that you are here, I ask you to stick with me as we take your self-discovery journey together. I promise to make our time together valuable and worthwhile.

In the pages ahead, you will find some areas of information and practices more helpful than others - and that is great! I encourage you to apply what works best for you. You will benefit from the knowledge that you gain and the ensuing exciting transformation of character.

Enjoy!

Table of Contents

Foreword

Self-confidence is attractive. It is a virtue every champion possesses. Whether it is Rosa Parks or Martin Luther King Junior, every household name possesses a striking belief in their abilities that makes them outstanding. It makes you a natural leader because people always need someone to inspire them, and give them the courage to find their voice during challenging periods.

In *Ruling Your World,* Paul reminds us all that we are kings and queens who will never be acknowledged unless we perceive ourselves as royalty and sacred. He shows us the inner beauty and glory we all possess via our uniqueness that must be sharpened, expressed, and reinvented to make us whole.

The world awaits your manifestation but it will never happen when and if you doubt yourself. Self-doubt can be so destructive that it can prevent you from ever-widening your horizon and seeing beyond your current circumstances. You are a king or queen and your life is your kingdom. This is the book you need to inculcate a winning mentality that will inspire everyone around you.

Introduction

J. M. Barrie

You are a force of nature but you will never discover your true power until you start believing in yourself. We live in a world where people do their best to shut us up so that we will never realize the greatness that lies within us. In the Bible story of Joseph, his brothers and even his father rebuked him for speaking about his dreams. They could not imagine that he would be greater than they were.

There will always be people who are afraid of your success. Some people benefit from the fact that they live a lowly and subservient life. They offer you peanuts to keep you in penury and servitude because it somehow makes them feel better about themselves. The moment you make any step toward achieving greatness, they will try to stop you.

The good news is that no force on earth is strong enough to stop you as long as you don't shoot yourself in the foot. Self-confidence opens the door to self-development, which eventually leads to self-actualization. You were born a giant, don't die a dwarf! I am so excited to get started with you on this journey that will train you and help you to develop your self-esteem and self-worth! Today is a good day!

Chapter One:
Dear Eagle, Fly!

"Believe you can and you are halfway there."

Theodore Roosevelt

Some years ago, I applied for a job in a private secondary school. It was a job I simply wanted as an additional means of income because I depended more on professional writing to pay my bills. Surprisingly, I saw many individuals who were working in this school full-time as their means of sustenance and paying their bills. I struggled to understand how they were able to manage themselves on such meager salaries.

Whenever they were paid their salaries, they would kowtow in appreciation to the boss of the company. I knew I couldn't stay there for long but how many people limited themselves to such low-paying jobs did not leave my mind. I realized that the difference between many of the staff of that school and me was our mindset.

I was so extremely confident in my abilities that the boss of the school felt intimidated the first day she met me. I knew I was going places and the value I have for my abilities can be quite scary. Nonetheless, I always do all I can to avoid pride and arrogance because there is a thin line between self-confidence and cockiness.

You Are An Eagle

Eagles are majestic birds that dominate the sky. By exploring some of the attributes of eagles, we will begin this journey:

They Are The Symbol Of Freedom And Peace

Freedom and peace are crucial in life but only a few people possess these qualities. Peace comes from a genuine feeling of satisfaction with your life but you can never have it unless you are doing the right things. Personal growth and progress will make you happier and will help you to enjoy inner tranquility. Low self-esteem is linked to a perception of stagnancy. When you do not feel that you are making progress and doing your best to fulfill your potential, low self-worth is a natural response.

The world will always do its best to cage you. Structures are created for the sake of organization and uniqueness. However, they tend to restrict people who have great abilities.

Do not restrict yourself to the perception and vision of people around you. Financial stability and independence will only come to you when you discover yourself and pursue your dreams. It all begins by believing that you can write your name in gold. Take bold steps and dare to be different. Respect is never just given. You have to earn it.

They Are Visionary

How do you see yourself? Your perception of yourself will determine whether you will scale new heights or live the rest of your life in oblivion. Indeed, family background plays a crucial role in our success and ambitions. Some people have a higher chance of achieving success in life because of the hard work and reputation of their families. If you are a member of the royal family of England, for example, three square meals a day will never be one of your worries. Life can be so unfair and you have to deal with it.

Complaining about the inequality that exists in life will not change anything. Instead, you should be more concerned about how you can make the best out of your life despite the challenges and obstacles. Beyond your current state, what kind of woman or man do you want to become? Do you deserve to be great? Your answers to this question will determine the kind of decisions you will make, which will eventually determine your fate. The fact that you were born in a manger does not mean that you cannot become the king of kings!

They Are Expert Hunters

Eagles are hunters and they are professionals in this respect. Building your self-esteem demands that you sharpen your skills. What can you offer? What do you know how to do? Can you write, speak, build, teach, develop websites, or treat people? Whatever it is that you do, you must work assiduously to become the best. Whenever people are looking for the best in your field, your name should be there. Invest in yourself. Train and retrain yourself. Attend seminars, buy books, ask questions from your superiors, and never stop learning.

Whenever people meet you after some time, it should be evident that you have moved a notch higher. When you are highly professional, you will not need adverts. Your work will speak for you. Your company will feel privileged to have you as an employee. Management will be afraid to lose you. A friend told me of how his boss increased his salary each time he informed her that he wanted to leave the organization, which was three times! Meanwhile, some other people who tried to leave the company were allowed to go. You can confidently ask for a pay rise when you know you offer value.

They Have A Kingly Mindset

Eagles rule the sky and they flaunt it. They are powerful and dominant. It is never best to settle for crumbs when you have the potential to buy the bakery. I once offered a person the opportunity to earn more money through freelancing but he rather wanted a 9 to 5 job that would not get him even half of what he could earn by freelancing. It is more and more obvious to me that many people are mentally caged.

They have the mindset of a freed slave who prefers the security of being fed by his former master to the freedom of working to earn his own money. There are many people ready to exploit you when you do not know your worth. Dear eagle, the world has myriads of wonderful opportunities waiting for people who know their worth and know what they want. You are a king or queen and no one should tell you otherwise. You might not rule the world but you should rule your world. The days of living a lowly and caged life are over. It is time to fly and rule the sky!

They Have A Strong Grip

Eagles are always in control and no one can take away whatever they are holding from them. Many people allow circumstances to determine the quality of life they live. The fact that you are currently an immigrant or refugee does not mean that you cannot rise above the situation. Your past does not determine your future. Rather, your future is a product of the decisions you make today. Your future is as beautiful as your current investments. Quit blaming the government or anyone else for your circumstances.

It is time to have a strong grip on your life. You are in control and you have the power to rewrite your story even when you have endured a torrid past. No other person has the right to determine your life but you. The days of grumbling and complaining are over. Many people are counting on you. It is time to start making courageous decisions. Your story can become an inspiration to others in the future if only you make up your mind to turn things around. Dear eagle, fly!

Chapter Two: Become Your Exorcist Of Fear

"To overcome fear is the quickest way to gain your self-confidence."

Roy T. Bennett

It is normal to be afraid of failing again, especially if you have failed in the past. The humiliation that came from your previous failures will always threaten to prevent you from trying again. Nonetheless, this is a demon you need to exorcise as soon as possible. This chapter offers you tips that will enable you to deal with fear and trauma to improve the quality of your life.

The Bliss Of A New Beginning

Don't waste your energy trying to change opinions... Do your thing, and don't care if they like it."

Tina Fey

Many people want to be given a second chance when they fail but do not want to allow others to atone for their failures. Mason Greenwood was only a teenager but he was shining brightly. It was obvious that he was the next big thing for Manchester United and England. He could shoot with both feet and was already a nightmare of nightmares, albeit being a teenager. The world was at his feet and it was only a matter of time before he began to set records.

However, just when no one thought anything could go wrong, disaster struck. An unfortunate recording and image of his alleged assault on his girlfriend was the last thing anyone expected to see in the media. It was a sad day for his fans and the fans of Manchester United. It was a disgrace and he was rightfully removed from the squad. Could this be the end of a star that had only just started shining? Many hoped he would rot in jail while some hoped he would stage a comeback and redeem himself.

When news broke that he was added to the Manchester United squad some months after the unfortunate incident, tongues were wagging and it was obvious that many people didn't want him to be given another chance. Yet, it is certain that many of those individuals would plead to be given a second chance if they had messed up. This is the reality of the world we live in. Many people are hypocrites who want a second chance but would be the most vocal antagonists when others are allowed to redeem themselves.

Therefore, do not let it grieve or shock you when no one believes you can recover after a setback. Sadly, it is the people closest to us that discourage us the most, sometimes. However, do not let fear stop you from trying again, regardless of what has happened in the past. You can cast out the demon of fear by trying to clip your wings in the following ways:

Learn From The Past

If you don't learn from your mistakes, you are only planning to fail again. You cannot successfully stage a comeback unless you have insight into the reasons your previous attempt was not successful. Why did your last relationship fail? Why were you sacked in your previous role? What were the factors responsible for your previous business or investment failures? Failure to objectively evaluate past mistakes is the reason some people find themselves in the same pit all over again.

You are not honest with yourself when you try again, simply because you want to prove others wrong. This is the reason some people start a new relationship almost immediately after a heartbreak. They want to prove to their ex that they can find another person. In the long run, they end the relationship again. Avoid the trap of proving a point to anyone. Your life is a personal story you should write without pressure from others.

Improve Yourself

When you discover the reasons you failed earlier, it is recommended that you equip yourself with the necessary knowledge and skills that will prepare you for your next attempt. When a military operation fails, the next logical step is to acquire the kind of ammunition that will enhance the success of the next operation. It is easier to know how you can improve yourself when you objectively evaluate your previous attempt.

Find books and connect to a mentor that can help you with the loopholes that prevented you from succeeding the previous time. It is good that you have the desire to bounce back after a setback but it is useless to do the same things with the same technique and expect things to be different. Persistence, without a willingness to improve, is a reckless attempt to waste your time and destroy your self-esteem.

Create A Plan

After you have improved yourself and equipped yourself with the necessary skills that will enable you to succeed, it is time to formulate a plan. Of course, your plan will be different because you are more experienced and fortified. Many times, the reason some people make quality decisions is because of their previous failures. So, your mistakes in the past are added ammunition if you know how to use them wisely.

Let your plan reflect your experience. Your mistakes help you to be aware of approaches that will not work. For example, if your previous investment failed because you didn't do your research about the business, your new plan will involve studying the market dynamics and pathways of the business in your next attempt. You are wiser now because you have failed in the past.

Find Sources Of Inspiration

It is okay to be scared that you might fail again after a setback. Even when you have a better plan, you might be wondering if it is nothing but another failed attempt. Nonetheless, you can never make progress unless you try. If you are struggling to believe in yourself after a setback, find the stories of people who have been in similar situations. It helps to know that there have been people who have gone through the same path but achieved success despite unfavorable circumstances.

It is always better when you know such people around you. It makes it easier to ask them questions rather than make assumptions. Their words of encouragement will boost your morale and convince you that you can also turn things around as they did. You can join an online community when you don't have such people around you.

Take Concrete Steps

You have not done anything until you have taken concrete steps to get it done. Every plan is wonderful on paper until tested. In football, matches are not won by the team that has the best players on paper. In the same way, you will not achieve anything until you try. Whatever it is you need to do should be done without wasting time.

It is okay to take your time to equip yourself with the knowledge and skills you need to succeed in your next attempt. Nonetheless, do not use that excuse to procrastinate. Whoever is trying and failing is better than the person who is only a spectator. The person who is failing is acquiring experiences that will eventually lead to success. So, it is better to fail than to do nothing. If you try, you might fail or succeed but if you do not make any attempt, your failure is sealed and stamped.

Chapter Three:
Dissecting Self-Doubt

"As soon as you trust yourself, you will know how to live."

Johann Wolfgang von Goethe

Self-doubt is cancerous. It keeps you in a cocoon that guarantees that you will struggle to achieve greatness. Therefore, you must be deliberate about dealing with low self-esteem to restore your confidence. This chapter will handle the possible reasons you doubt yourself.

Why Do People Experience Low Self-Esteem

Based on research and anecdotal evidence, below are some of the reasons people experience self-doubt:

A Harsh Upbringing

Parents typically love to exert themselves on their children. They are symbols of authority in the home and they always want to be in charge.

However, in some cases, they can be overbearing. Children can be silly and they always need guidance. They always need the help of older people to help them make quality decisions. Nonetheless, parents must be empathetic and patient with their children to avoid ruining their self-esteem.

Research has proven that children with problematic childhoods tend to grow into broken adults. Therefore, a close watch might help you to discover that your lack of self-esteem is due to the kind of upbringing you had. If your parents were always harsh and always compared you with others, you might struggle to believe in yourself as an adult. The moment you discover the source of the problem, it is half solved. Be deliberate about uprooting the seeds of low self-esteem that were sown in your life as a child, to change your mentality as an adult.

Previous Failures

No one wants to fail because no one wants to be associated with failure. When a person is successful, they have many friends. People are always around them because of the things they can gain from them. On the other hand, people who are perceived as failures and losers rarely have friends. In some cases, even their family members stay away from them. Previous failures are the easiest ways for your self-esteem to be shattered.

It gets worse when you fail even though you thought you had a perfect plan. If you have been cocky during the process and didn't allow anyone to offer you advice or suggestions, it can be lonely and you might struggle to recover from it. You might have made a lot of enemies for yourself during that period, which might make it almost insurmountable to recover from the setback.

Self-Criticism

Normally, you should demand a lot from yourself because it is necessary to achieve tangible success in life. It is expected that you put yourself under pressure to enable you to fulfill your potential. However, it can be problematic when you always find a way to put yourself down whenever you make a mistake. Indeed, you should set a standard for the kind of performance you expect from yourself but you can never be perfect as a human being.

Life will not always give you what you want. There will always be days of imperfection. So, it is not the best approach to always criticize yourself. When self-criticism is at its peak, it will make you incapable of enjoying your success. You will always look down on your achievements when you have this mindset. Self-critics are fond of upward and downward social comparison, which makes them always feel that they are not doing enough regardless of their success, which eventually takes its toll on their self-esteem.

Unforgiveness

A combination of previous failures and self-criticism can make it difficult for you to forgive yourself when you make mistakes. Some people can hate themselves for life for certain things they didn't do right at some point in their lives. This is not the best approach because it will always drain your self-esteem and make you ridicule yourself.

"It's not an easy journey to get to a place where you forgive people but it is such a powerful place because it frees you."

Tyler Perry

It is never easy to let go of the past, especially when you make decisions that cost you heavily. Nonetheless, it is the only solution. Self-doubt will make you a shadow of your former self. It will keep you in one spot and make it challenging for you to move forward in life. It will ridicule your previous achievements and make it appear as though you were just lucky to succeed in the past.

Lack Of Self-Development

Naturally, you will feel stagnant when you are not developing yourself and this will eventually affect your self-esteem. Life changes rapidly and you might discover that you are already left behind in no time if you are not updating yourself with new knowledge and skills. When you are not improving, others will move past you and it will speed up the rate of feeling irrelevant.

Every organization wants productive people and you might be demoted or sacked when you do not meet the standards. Younger and newer people might become the leader of your team and this will hurt you. It will make you feel irrelevant and this will affect your self-worth. You will have no one to blame but yourself when this happens to you. So, if you notice that you struggle with self-confidence, you need to question your commitment to improving yourself.

Negative Aura

A negative attitude will ruin your self-esteem. When you have a culture of expecting nothing from life, the chances are low that you will take reasonable steps to improve the quality of your life. Some people claim they are being realistic by employing a pessimistic approach to life. They claim that they expect nothing to avoid disappointments. Of course, this sounds like a logical precautionary measure but it will make you struggle to strive for excellence.

Nothing is ever guaranteed in life but it is less likely when you do not approach life with optimism. Research has established a link between optimism and self-esteem. Pessimistic people are likely to experience low self-esteem while optimistic people are likely to have high self-worth. Regardless of what has happened in the past, it is not recommended to carry a negative presence because it will make others avoid you. No one wants to be around people who only see challenges and not opportunities.

Presence Of Negative People

The kind of people you have around you determines your perception of life. If you have people who see themselves as victims of circumstances around you, the chances are high that you will generally have a pessimistic view of life. Instead of yearning for success, you will blame others for not giving you a fair crack.

Negative people also tend to make it difficult for you to recover from a setback.

Whenever you try to move forward, they will remind you of how you failed previously and this will get you stuck in one position. The success of others will annoy you and you will always be suspicious of others, which will make people want to stay away from you.

Chapter Four:
Symptoms Of Self-Doubt

"Once we believe in ourselves, we can risk curiosity, wonder, spontaneous delight, or any experience that reveals the human spirit."

E. E. Cummings

Just like a medical doctor, you can run a diagnosis to know if you are suffering from self-doubt. There are certain symptoms associated with low self-esteem. When you see them, you can tell that you need to work on your self-confidence. This chapter will discuss these signs.

Diagnosing Self-Doubt

It is possible to detect low self-esteem through keen observation. The following symptoms are linked to self-doubt:

Desperation

People with low self-esteem are usually desperate. When they are given an opportunity, they always do all they can to keep it even to their detriment. When such people are in relationships, they are usually clingy and full of insecurities. They tend to suspect their partners because they feel that the person might be attracted to someone better than them. If you observe this pattern of behavior in your life, it is time to do something about it.

It will make you less desirable to your partner because no one wants to be in a relationship with a person that does not trust them. When people who have self-doubt are told by their partners that they do not want to be in the relationship anymore, they will be desperate to hold on because they are scared that they might never be able to find another relationship that is worth it again.

Fear Of Failure

Fear of failure is real and many people deal with it but it is at another level when it comes to people with self-doubt. They are so afraid of failing that they prefer to do nothing rather than make an attempt. Meanwhile, you are guaranteed to live a low life when you are not willing to take risks. People with low self-esteem always avoid leaving their comfort zone because they are usually afraid of the unknown.

Such people see challenges in every situation rather than the possibility it offers them to improve the quality of their lives. When such individuals have the opportunity to study in another country that offers a higher level of quality in terms of infrastructure and facilities than their home nation, they will rather be concerned about the language barrier and the difficulties that come with settling in a new place. They will rather stay with their current friends who have little to offer them than try to explore new opportunities that offer better possibilities.

A Reactive Approach To Life

People with low self-esteem hardly have plans. Consequently, they are hardly prepared for the future, which often makes them victims of circumstances. Such people usually get stranded because they never think about other options whenever they are enjoying a current situation. While working, they never make plans for their retirement until it is almost too late. Such people are fond of making decisions at the very end.

When they are trusted with projects, they never make concrete plans to get them done. They end up procrastinating until the deadline is close, sometimes because they feel the task is too challenging. They are not confident in their ability to succeed in tasks before they tackle them. In psychology, this is known as self-efficacy. Studies have linked low self-esteem to low self-efficacy. Such individuals are usually behind in their schedules and hardly showcase any form of efficiency and organization.

Mediocrity

It is easy to spot a person with low self-esteem. By simply looking at the way they dress and speak, you can spot that they lack confidence in their ability. Sadly, there are predators in this business world who will readily take advantage of such individuals. They will offer them pay way below what they generally offer and those people will happily take it because they think that is what they deserve.

Such individuals have been wired to think that they have to work extremely hard to achieve financial stability. The truth is that you can always acquire a high-level skill that will enable you to earn more without working as hard as some people. Some people will pay you more when you can offer knowledge and consultancy instead of working a menial job that offers little. However, people with low self-esteem give up quickly on themselves and will rather stick with low-paying jobs than invest in themselves to increase their ability to earn more.

Purposeless Living

Goal setting is linked to high self-esteem. It takes self-confidence to set goals and work towards achieving them. This is never the case with people with low self-esteem. They rarely have short-term and long-term goals. Even when they set targets, they are usually short-term ones. They hardly have visions of becoming great because of their lack of confidence in their ability. Consequently, they have nothing they are truly living for.

They only live in the moment, flowing with the tides, and following bandwagons. Such people hardly have a sense of uniqueness and individuality. They are quick to jump on any trend and participate in all sorts of ridiculous challenges on social media. Anyone can hire them and ask them to do things for money because they have no plans for their lives. They get involved in dangerous and damaging activities such as drug and alcohol abuse to fight off the feeling of worthlessness they usually have.

Instability

Stability is linked to goal setting. When a person has plans for their life, they know what they want, which makes them selective in the kind of things they do. They know that everyone cannot be their friend and spouse. When a person lacks self-esteem, they readily accept the friendship of anyone who tries to come into their lives. They never create boundaries, opening the door for all sorts of people to find their way into their lives.

Consequently, they are usually unstable in their choices and commitments. They hardly work any job for long because they tend to accept offers without verifying or reviewing the details of what their role in the organization entails. They usually find out that they cannot cope and will eventually opt out and start looking for a new role. They hardly have job satisfaction due to their tendency to accept employment opportunities hastily.

Pessimism

Pessimism is linked to low self-esteem. People with self-doubt generally do not expect good things to happen to them. Whenever they have a setback, they find it challenging to recover because they hardly believe in their ability to turn things around. Consequently, they tend to take rash steps such as suicidal attempts because they often throw in the towel easily. Such people usually need the support of others to cope because they cannot be trusted to handle themselves.

When they are around you, they are often unnecessarily cautious. Whenever people are making plans to achieve something great, they are usually the first to point out the challenges. Indeed, it is important to make an objective evaluation of your chances in life. Nonetheless, a little bit of optimism is not a bad idea.

Chapter Five:
Perks Of High Self-Esteem

"Why should I care what other people think of me? I am who I am and who I wanna be."

Avril Lavigne

Research has established a link between high self-esteem and well-being. Low self-esteem will ruin your psychological well-being. It is linked to anxiety and depression. No one wants to be associated with people with low self-worth because they often carry a negative presence. On the other hand, high self-esteem has several advantages. This chapter will list and discuss them.

The Benefits Of Building Self-Confidence

When you have high self-esteem, below are some of the advantages you stand to enjoy:

Pursuit of Greatness

Optimism is linked to high self-esteem. A confident individual is certain that they have what it takes to succeed in life and they pursue their dreams. In some cases, some people predict how far they will go in life and they make it happen. The reality is that there is no dream that is beyond your reach as long as you believe in yourself. Even when no one in your family or nation has ever achieved certain feats, that does not mean they are out of bonds for you.

In every nation, there is always the first person to achieve a particular feat. Whether it is in politics, sports, education, or technology, there will always be the first person from a country to reach certain milestones. When Tobi Amusan of Nigeria broke the world record in the 110-meter hurdles race in 2022, she was the first Nigerian to break a world record at that time. You can always get to heights beyond your imagination with self-confidence and hard work. Every superstar emerged with the determination that they could achieve greatness.

Focus

When you believe in yourself, you will keep pursuing greatness even if no one believes in you. The path to success can be cumbersome and full of obstacles, which makes it available to only the individuals that are willing to pay the price. Self-confidence is an essential ingredient in your journey to success. It has been linked to focusing. The fact that you believe in your ability to succeed will help you to keep going, especially during dark days. There will always be days of setbacks when it looks as though your dreams will not come true.

Every champion experiences moments when it seems all hope is lost and every potential winner will go through this phase. It is your confidence in yourself that will keep you going during this period. Do not be perturbed when some of the people you love and trust do not believe in you. At some point, my teacher in college did not believe I could be accepted by one of the best schools in my country but I believed in myself and achieved it. It was a shock to most people who knew me but that is the power of self-belief.

Harmonious Romantic Relationships

People with low self-esteem are likely to find themselves in abusive relationships due to their desperation. The fact that they do not believe that they deserve to be loved and respected makes it easy for them to fall into the wrong hands. On the other hand, people with high self-worth know their value, which makes them selective in their approach to choosing a romantic partner. The fact that a person loves you and professes their love to you is not enough reason to accept being a partner to that person.

In the same way, you cannot work for every company that wants to acquire your talent, so you cannot become the partner of every man or woman who claims to love you. Self-confidence will make you patient until you have found the kind of man or woman you want. You do not have to endure your marriage out of desperation. Do not settle for less than the best. It is better not to marry than to be married to the wrong person.

Quality Interpersonal Relationships

Sadly, our friends and families can take us for granted sometimes. When you have low self-worth, you can settle for anything and accept anything. Such people never make demands in their relationships with others because they do not want to offend anyone. Indeed, it is not recommended that you place unreasonable demands on others. Nonetheless, you should let your friends and families know what you want because it is impossible to please a person who does not state clearly what they want.

Many relationships are ruined because the people involved are not willing to have open, honest discussions about their needs. Let your friends know what hurts you so that they can avoid it. When you do not use this approach, you become vulnerable to being hurt by others and it might not be deliberate. So, it is in your best interest to be confident enough to make demands in your relationships to avoid getting hurt by the people you care about. It is also good that you ask your loved ones what they want, to avoid friction in your relationship with them.

Robust Professional Relationships

Why should you work at a job that does not make you happy? Sadly, this is the reality for many people. Studies have shown that many people in the US are not happy with their jobs. It is understood that many individuals only work to make ends meet. The moment you only work to earn money, you are inadvertently a slave. You should be able to wake up in the morning and feel delighted that you are going to work. However, you will never experience this feeling when you pick up whatever role is available to you.

Self-confident people have a knack for working jobs they are passionate about. Of course, this is not easy but it is possible. Even if the job that pays your bills is not your number one passion, it should be something you are proud of. When you are not happy with your professional life, it can take a toll on your private life. Besides, you cannot be at your best when you are in a role that does not make you happy.

Fulfillment And Personal Satisfaction

The combination of all the aforementioned perks of self-confidence will help you to live the happy and fulfilled life you deserve. Self-actualization is the height of human experience, according to psychologists. It is the zone where you feel complete and accomplished. It is a combination of a quality romantic relationship, top-notch interpersonal relationships, and excellent professional relationships. There is no way you will not be happy with your life when you are satisfied with your marital life, interpersonal relationships, and career.

Throw a meaningful spiritual life into the mix and you will be cooking and eating a gourmet dish! The issue most times is that many people are not aware of all the great things and beautiful life they can have when they dare to believe in themselves. You are a king or queen and no one should change your identity. You might not rule at Buckingham Palace but no one can deny you your rightful place on the throne of your world. You only live once; enjoy it to the fullest by building your confidence.

Chapter Six:
How To Overcome
Self-Doubt

"A diamond doesn't start out polished and shining. It once was nothing special but with enough pressure and time, it becomes something spectacular. I'm that diamond."

Solange Nicole

The fact that you have reasons to doubt your ability to succeed is a sign that you are a human being. You have things that scare you sometimes and that is perfectly normal. Nonetheless, it is evident that self-doubt is limiting because it will hinder you from fulfilling your potential. Therefore, you must discover ways to overcome it. You will find useful tips in this regard in this chapter.

Defeating Self-Doubt

Overcoming self-doubt and low self-esteem take deliberate effort and commitment. The following tips can help you in this respect:

Shun Perfectionism

Perfectionism has been linked to various psychological dysfunctions. It is an attribute that can make you struggle with your self-worth. Perfectionists are never satisfied and struggle to practice gratitude. Even when others are appreciating their efforts, they struggle to feel the same way. This mindset can make you struggle to enjoy your success and growth. You will be unhappy simply because everything does not look perfect. It is in your best interest to avoid this approach to life because it will take its toll on your self-worth.

Overcome The Fear Of Failure

The fact is, the majority of great heroes failed many times in their discoveries before they attained the level of success that they desired. Even though they failed, they never stopped working on their vision till they reached the level of success they wanted. One way to overcome the fear of failure is not to be afraid of it.

One of the most powerful weapons to overcome the fear of failure is to have a clear positive vision of where you are going and be ready to take the necessary steps to reach your destination because determination toward both success and failure begins in the heart.

Discover Your Strengths

We all have unique strengths. When defined and nurtured, we can live out our best lives for ourselves and in the service of others. Strengths aren't the same as talents because they can be developed. You will have a better chance of succeeding when you identify your strengths. Be conscious of what is going on within and around you. Within means seeing ourselves and becoming aware of our thoughts, feelings, desires, and passion.

Also, note the things that give you joy. Watch out for that need your heart is crying out to be seen in the world of humanity. Meanwhile, the things going on around us, refer to how other people view us, our strengths, behaviors, and reactions. Our strengths lie between the deep desire of our hearts and the needs that are yet to be met around us.

Have a clear, positive vision about where you are going. Imagining how life will be after you have reached your goal is a great motivator to keep you moving forward. Guide your heart with diligence and the necessary information that will help you fulfill the vision of your heart. Set goals that you know you are capable of achieving. Taking one small step at a time will help build your confidence, keep you moving forward, and prevent you from getting overwhelmed with visions of your final goal.

Admit Your Limitations

We need to admit our limitations in life because if we fail to admit our limitations, the same weakness will keep repeating itself over and over again. Every person within themselves is limited because a single tree does not make a forest. So, we must recognize fully that a single person cannot fulfill a vision in their heart. A vision can be given to a single person but it will take the contribution of many to bring the vision to fulfillment. This is the beauty of vision. It makes room for others to find their relevance in it.

Knowing this will build self-confidence in you and the life of those around you because everyone will be able to see his or her relevance. If you act like you can do everything alone, you're going to find it quite humiliating when you fail miserably in front of everyone. On this note, we should admit that we need the help of those who have gone ahead and the help of our core colleagues and those who are coming after us.

To grow in life, and as a leader, one needs to welcome criticism with an open mind.

Mask Or Work On Your Limitations

It is very crucial that in knowing our limitations, we consciously work on them. Not only should we believe in our ability which is good, but let us also trust and believe in the ability of others, in the light of our pursuit of building self-confidence. Whether you are a leader or not, one person can't know everything, and acceptance of this is key to embracing humility. Always be open to accepting others' opinions and asking for their expertise, when required. Embracing different viewpoints when your own may be limited, gives you a better perspective.

We must know that criticism is not for our destruction but rather for building us up. For if we are going to fully build our self-confidence, criticism is a stage we must pass through just like the way raw gold must pass through the fire. So, whenever criticism comes, let us not forget to rejoice and stay focused because they are all working together for our good.

Make New Friends

Self-confidence cannot be built in idleness or isolation. This is because it requires both you and the kind of people that surround you. Every dream or vision needs the support of others because we are all given unique and special abilities so that we can know and recognize the value and place of each of us in developing self-confidence and achieving success in every sphere of life.

There is nothing new under the sun; what every person needs in one phase of their lives, has been made available to another individual. This is why having the right association is paramount if we are going to build our self-confidence. Making new friends in the light of our dream is very important because it is impossible to succeed alone. So, the kind of friends we make, determines how far we will go in building our self-confidence. Let us make friends in the light of our pursuit.

Chapter Seven:
Maintaining Self-Confidence

"Public opinion is a weak tyrant compared with our own private opinion."

Henry David Thoreau

It is fantastic to build and regain confidence but the truth is that you can lose it somewhere along the line. Confidence is not a permanent attribute people possess. Even the most confident human beings have bad days when they lose confidence in themselves. Therefore, you must learn how to maintain your self-esteem. You will find valuable tips that can help you in this area throughout this chapter.

Things Can Change

You are a human being and this reality implies that you are not infallible. Things can change quickly. Once upon a time, Jose Mourinho was the darling of the football world. He announced himself to the world when he won the UEFA Champions League with FC Porto as the underdog in the 2003/2004 season. Many clubs across Europe wanted him as their manager.

Everyone wanted to be the proud owner of this upcoming master tactician. It was obvious that Porto would not be able to hold on to him anymore and it was not surprising when he signed for Chelsea FC the following season.

With the ambition of the owner, Roman Abramovich, it appeared like a match made in heaven. Mourinho announced himself as the "Special One" and he lived up to his nickname as he went on to win two Premier League titles with Chelsea despite the presence of world-class coaches such as the legendary Sir Alex Ferguson of Manchester United and Arsene Wenger of Arsenal FC. It seems he could do no wrong but things soon went sour and his marriage with the club came to an end in 2007 after it appeared he was losing in the dressing room and results were beginning to get worse.

In 2020, Thomas Tuchel, a German football tactician, became the manager of Chelsea FC in the middle of the season. The club was struggling under former manager, Frank Lampard before his arrival and it appeared that he was only brought in to steady the ship. However, he overachieved in his first season when he won the UEFA Champions League to the surprise of many. It appeared as though

Chelsea had finally found a manager for the long haul.

He followed that success with a UEFA Super Cup and a Club World Cup in the next season. These were trophies that the club had never won in its history. He also took the club to the final of the Carabao Cup and the FA Cup. Fast-forward to September 2022, he was sacked after just seven games into the season. These stories show that things can change no matter how wonderful they have been. So, the fact that your confidence is sky high at the moment does not mean that it cannot take a nosedive when some unpredictable event takes place.

How To Maintain Self-Confidence

Since things can grow worse, including your confidence, you must work deliberately at maintaining it. The following tips can guide you in this respect:

Admit That Things Can Change

People lose confidence in themselves when they do not have a realistic view of life. Some individuals expect things to continue the way they are only to be given the shock of their lives. Some people are privileged to have successful parents but their lives took a nosedive when their parents died unexpectedly. They had been wasteful before that time because they thought things would never change.

Consequently, their confidence levels crash after that and some never recover from the incident. Life is as volatile as the stock market. My dad would always say that life is a combination of a little sweetness and a little bitterness. Once you are conversant with and convinced of this reality, the bad days will never make you give up on yourself.

Stay Around Confident People

We cannot overemphasize the importance of the impact of the kind of people you have around you. If you have people that give up easily around you, the chances are high that you will struggle to develop resilience. On the other hand, if you tend to give up easily, your association with mentally strong people will help you to improve in this area. Therefore, one of the best ways you can develop and maintain self-confidence is by staying around individuals with high self-esteem.

Never Stop Learning

Learning new things has a way of improving your sense of self-worth. On the other hand, when you find out that there are many things you don't know, it dampens your morale. It gets worse when you are around people that like to make others feel bad when they realize that they are more knowledgeable than them. Therefore, it is essential that you continue to spend time learning and developing yourself. Have the habit of randomly checking something you are ignorant of. No knowledge is lost. Whenever you have the opportunity to educate others about something you know, you will feel better about yourself.

Practice Gratitude

One of the reasons people lose confidence in themselves is that they lack an attitude of gratitude. Perfectionism often gives birth to this syndrome. Therefore, to maintain your self-esteem and self-worth, have a culture of appreciating the things you have. Avoid comparing your achievement to the success of others because there will always be people whose achievements dwarf yours. Be deliberate about gratitude. Create time to list out all the things you cherish and value in your life and you will realize that your heart will be filled with gladness. It is a quick way to improve your mood and dispel negative emotions.

Leverage Journaling

A deliberate attempt to maintain your self-confidence should inspire you to create time to write out your thoughts and plans for the future. This practice is known as journaling. Your journal is that friend you can always have around you even when traveling. It is a practice that is linked to happiness and high self-esteem.

The fact that you are willing to pick up a notepad and document your plans and achievements automatically ignites the feeling of importance in you. It raises your self-esteem and inspires you to strive to achieve more. Joining a community of people online that have this practice can also help you to practice it consistently because we can all lose track of productive activities.

Practice Meditation And Mindfulness

Meditation and mindfulness are not the same but they have the same purpose. They are activities that help to keep away negative emotions from you and give you the inner tranquility you desire. Meanwhile, keeping your mind free from limiting thoughts is an effective method of maintaining your self-confidence. You will need a place where you are not distracted, to practice meditation but you can practice mindfulness anywhere. It does not require a special outfit or place.

All you need to do to practice mindfulness is keep your mind on one thing at a time. It is a practice you can have while praying or even while dancing. The boisterous noise of a football match cannot even inhibit your mindfulness. In such a situation, all you need to do is to focus on the match and let nothing else bothers your mind.

Chapter Eight:
Building Confidence
In Others

"Self-confidence is Contagious."

Stephen Richard

We have spent most parts of this book discussing how you can build your confidence. We should spare this last chapter to discuss how you can inspire others to recover from setbacks.

Developing Other People's Self-Esteem

No one can become great without impacting others. Greatness is a product of the things we have achieved through our interaction with our fellow human beings. One of the best ways you can help other people in your circle or the ones far away from you is by helping them to believe in themselves. The following tips will help you in this endeavor:

Use Your Story

One of my secrets to success is the desire to inspire others with my story. I want to be able to tell others about how I achieved success despite the odds that were stacked against me. When helping others to overcome self-doubt, your story is an important weapon in your arsenal. People have more reasons to follow you and listen to it when they believe that you have been where they are.

You will naturally become the leader of such people. For example, if you have attempted suicide in the past but changed your mind and made the best out of your life, you are the natural mentor of people who ever had suicidal thoughts. In the same way, if you achieved success and have a good marriage after previously experiencing divorce, people who have been divorced will love to listen to you. They will willingly give you their hand to lead them out of your abyss into a glorious future.

Display Empathy

Empathy is observable and attractive. Some people make the mistake of helping others condescendingly. Some individuals are fond of posting about the people they help online to get cheap likes and engagement. It is appalling whenever I see people post about helping the less privileged on social media platforms. I keep wondering if they would have done the same if those people were their family members. Of course, it is not likely that they would have done the same if those people were individuals that they share close bonds.

It is not good to ridicule others simply because they need your help. Even if they did not come to your aid when you needed their help, that does not mean that you should shatter their self-confidence when they need you. The truth is that it is always a privilege to be able to contribute meaningfully to the lives of others. You might think that you are doing them a favor but a time will come in your life when you will be happy that you helped others. No one can experience fulfillment without contributing to the lives of others.

Be Realistic

When you meet people who need your help to regain their lives, you must be realistic. Avoid saying things that sound fanciful. For example, after a person has lost a job, it is pointless to tell such an individual that they can still become the president of the US. What is the point of that kind of information? Such motivation is only useful to a person that has just lost a presidential election.

Hillary Clinton would have been happy to hear you say something like that to her after she lost the presidential election. Ensure your words of encouragement do not sound like mockery to others. How can you do that? Ensure that you are sensitive to the situation of the person. Your words should be related to their current situation and not the fanciful dreams you create for them. If you fail to learn this skill, the people around you will not look forward to seeing you when they are experiencing challenges.

Prioritize Honesty

The people around you might have issues with your honesty toward them initially but they will eventually appreciate it. We all know the people who will tell us the truth and we eventually seek them out when we are ready to grow and improve. So, you mustn't tell people the things they want to hear but rather the truth. If a person has a setback due to a mistake they made, let them know without trying to make them feel guilty.

It is important to do this so that people can learn from their mistakes. Ensure that you point out to them that their past errors will not define their future. Nonetheless, a level of honesty is necessary for development and progress. If a person is not willing, to be honest with themselves, you should leave such people to themselves.

Point Out The Challenges

When people are in their lowest moments, they are usually desperate. Therefore, they are usually willing to take any lifeline you give them. Nonetheless, people must be aware of the challenges that come with every opportunity so that they do not give up somewhere along the line. Many individuals who introduce others to businesses that they claim can help them achieve financial stability are guilty of this.

Some people that introduce others to a business such as an affiliate marketing do not tell them about the challenges involved. Instead, they sell dreams to people. They claim it is a simple job to do and a person can quit their 9-5 job and travel around the world in a short time. This is not accurate and many people only find that out after they have sold their assets to buy courses from some of these online gurus. Let people know the sacrifices they will need to make to achieve success while helping them build or rebuild their self-esteem.

Offer Solutions

It is good to point out the mistakes people made that led to their problems. Nonetheless, it is more important to show them the way out. When you point out the errors of others without teaching them how to overcome them, you are only a cynical critic. Never criticize people you are not willing to help.

The world is full of such insensitive individuals who find joy in making others feel bad about themselves. You shouldn't join such people. What if you find out that you were part of an online mob contributing to the death of a person through suicide? Will you be happy with yourself then? Our world needs healing. It needs more rays of hope who will lovingly point out the mistakes of others and help them grow. The world is waiting for you!

Conclusion

Self-doubt is a trait that is common to all, even among the most confident of us. Fear comes because the realities of things around us are far from the things we desire to see and when the things that can be seen are giving us a picture of impossibility concerning unseen visions and dreams in our hearts.

This has been a wonderful, thrilling, and educational journey. While putting this material together, I was hoping that it would inspire millions of people around the world and help them to believe in themselves. If this book has had this impact on your life, then I have succeeded.

The different phases of life come with unique challenges that can shatter our confidence if care is not taken. You might have been broken by some of the experiences you had in the past but I am happy to announce that you have a glorious future, which you can access if only you consistently and genuinely believe in yourself.

When you suffer a setback, life will also give you opportunities to recover and grow. Sadly, some people do not leverage these chances. I am glad that you made it this far because it is a sign that you are committed to overcoming self-doubt and making the best of the beautiful parts of your life. You are unstoppable! Today is still a great day to be alive!

References

Pew Research. (2021, September 28). *3. How Americans view their jobs*. Pew Research Center's Social & Demographic Trends Project. Retrieved March 12, 2022, from https://www.pewresearch.org/social-trends/2016/10/06/3-how-americans-view-their-jobs/

Greenacre, Luke & Tung, N.M. & Chapman, Tom. (2014). Self-confidence, and the ability to influence. Academy of Marketing Studies Journal. 18. 169-180.

Reynolds CR, Richmond BO. What I think and feel: a revised measure of children's manifest anxiety. J Abnorm Child Psychol. 1978;6 (2):271–80.

Dittner AJ, Rimes K, Thorpe S. Negative perfectionism increases the risk of fatigue following a period of stress. Psychol Health 2010 Feb. [Accessed 17 October 2010]. Available from: http://www.informaworld.com/10.1080/08870440903225892.

Wang KT, Slaney RB, Rice KG. Perfectionism in Chinese university students from Taiwan: a study of psychological well-being and achievement motivation. Pers Individ Dif. 2007;42 (7):1279–90.

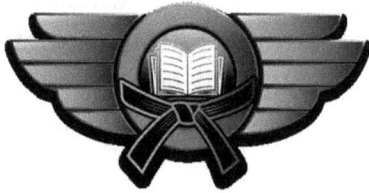

Thank you for reading this book!

If you found this book helpful, I would be grateful if you would **post an honest review on Amazon** so this book can reach other supportive readers like you!

All you need to do is digitally flip to the back and leave your review. Or visit amazon.com/author/senseipauldavid click the correct book cover and click on the blue link next to the yellow stars that say, "customer reviews."

As always...
It's a great day to be alive!

Get/Share Our FREE All-Ages Mental Health Book Now!

FREE Self-Development Book for Every Family

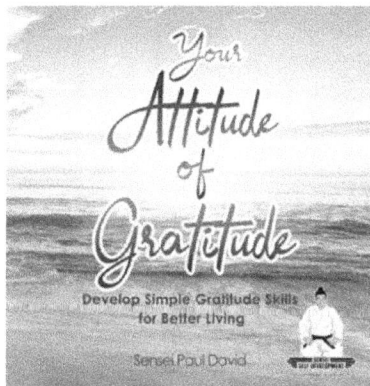

senseiselfdevelopment.senseipublishing.com

Click Below or Search Amazon for Another Book In This Series Or Visit:

www.amazon.com/author/senseipauldavid

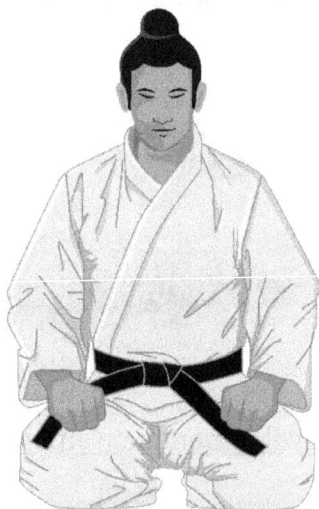

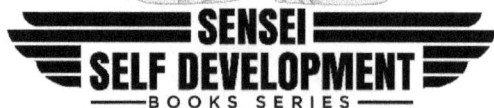

SENSEI
SELF DEVELOPMENT
BOOKS SERIES

senseiselfdevelopment.senseipublishing.com

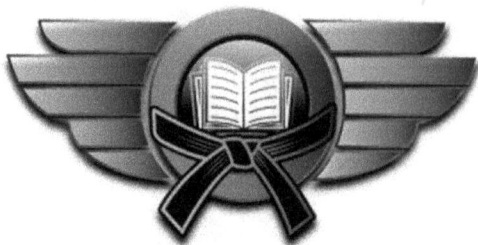

SENSEI PUBLISHING

It's A Great Day To Be Alive!

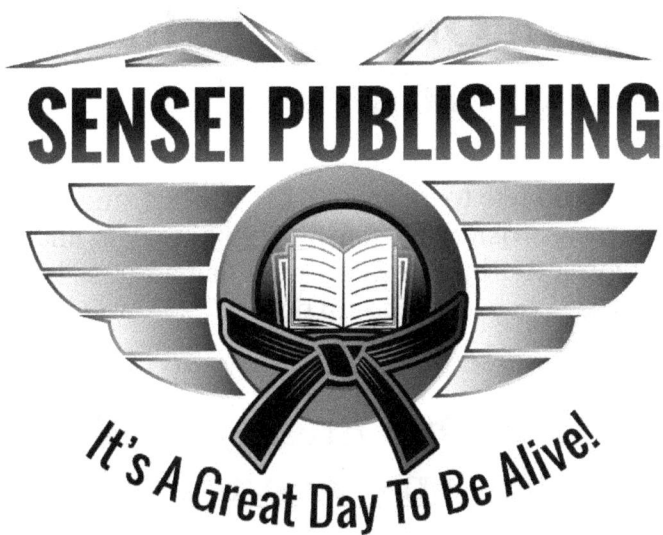

www.senseipublishing.com

@senseipublishing
#senseipublishing

Check out our **recommendations** for other books for adults & kids plus other great resources by visiting www.senseipublishing.com/resources/

Join Our Publishing Journey!

If you would like to receive FREE BOOKS, and special offers, please visit www.senseipublishing.com and join our newsletter by entering your email address in the pop-up box

Follow Our Engaging Blog NOW! senseipauldavid.ca

Get Our FREE Books Today!

Click & Share the Link Below

FREE Self-Development Book
senseiselfdevelopment.senseipublishing.com

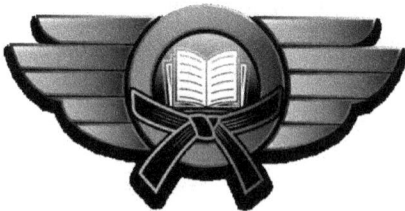

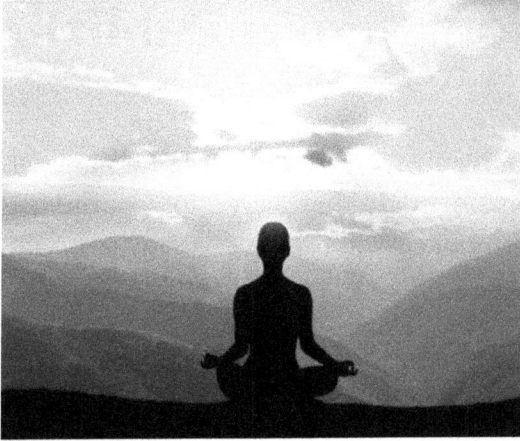

FREE BONUS!!!
Experience Over 25 FREE Engaging Guided
Meditations!

Prized Skills & Practices for Adults & Kids.
Help Restore Deep Sleep, Lower Stress,
Improve Posture, Navigate Uncertainty &
More.

Download the Free Insight Timer App and click the link
below:
http://insig.ht/sensei_paul

About Sensei Publishing

Sensei Publishing commits itself to helping people of all ages transform into better versions of themselves by providing high-quality and research-based self-development books with an emphasis on mental health and guided meditations. Sensei Publishing offers well-written e-books, audiobooks, paperbacks and online courses that simplify complicated but practical topics in line with its mission to inspire people towards positive transformation.

It's a great day to be alive!

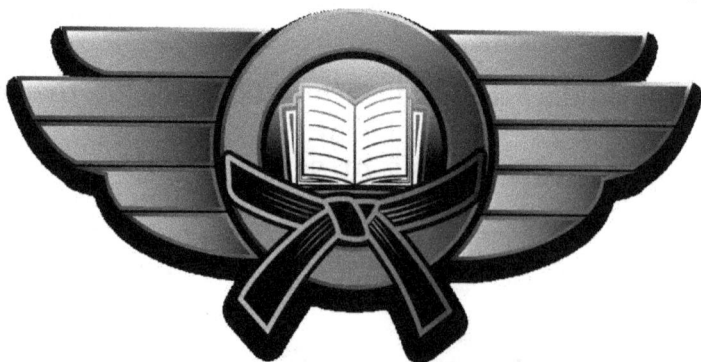

About the Author

I create simple & transformative eBooks & Guided Meditations for Adults & Children proven to help navigate uncertainty, solve niche problems & bring families closer together.

I'm a former finance project manager, private pilot, jiu-jitsu instructor, musician & former University of Toronto Fitness Trainer. I prefer a science-based approach to focus on these & other areas in my life to stay humble & hungry to evolve. I hope you enjoy my work and I'd love to hear your feedback.

- It's a great day to be alive!
Sensei Paul David

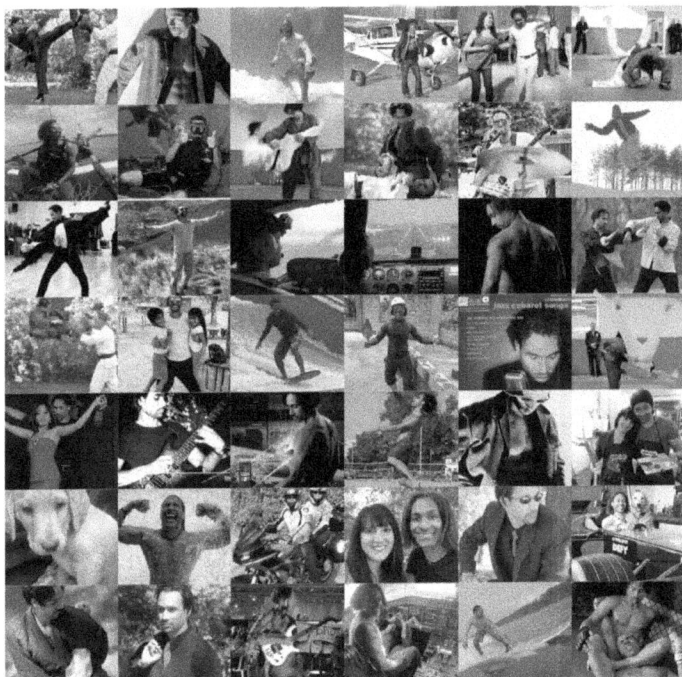

Scan & Follow/Like/Subscribe: Facebook, Instagram, YouTube: @senseipublishing

Scan using your phone/iPad camera for Social Media Visit us at www.senseipublishing.com and sign up for our newsletter to learn more about our exciting books and to experience our FREE Guided Meditations for Kids & Adults.

www.ingramcontent.com/pod-product-compliance
Lightning Source LLC
Chambersburg PA
CBHW060655030426
42337CB00017B/2622